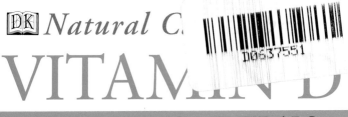

DK *Natural C...*
VITAMIN D

MAXIMIZING MINERALS

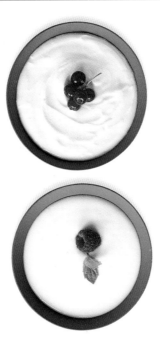

By STEPHANIE PEDERSEN

DORLING KINDERSLEY PUBLISHING, INC.

www.dk.com

CONTENTS

VITAMIN BASICS

The word "vitamin" is a relatively new term. The word first appeared in dictionaries in 1912 and was coined to describe the organic substances in food essential for most chemical processes in the body. Before vitamins were discovered, doctors recommended food itself: carrots (rich in vitamin A) to maintain vision, citrus fruit (high in vitamin C) to prevent scurvy, and whole grains and legumes (abundant in vitamin B_1) to ward off beriberi.

Scientists have identified 13 vitamins that are considered essential for health—essential because the body does not manufacture these nutrients itself. In other words, these vitamins must come either from food or from supplements. Essential vitamins are grouped into two categories: fat-soluble and water-soluble.

Essential fat-soluble vitamins include vitamins A, D, E, and K. These are stored in the body's fat to be used as needed. Because the body stockpiles fat-soluble vitamins, it is possible to take too much of one or more of these vitamins, although this rarely occurs. Vitamin overdose can lead to various symptoms, including headaches and irritability.

The essential water-soluble vitamins are C, B, B_1, B_2, B_3, B_5, B_6, B_{12}, folic acid, and biotin. These are not stored in the body: The body uses just what it needs at any given time and excretes the unused amount in the urine.

Two important points about vitamins. Many people believe that if they take nutritional supplements, they won't have to worry about a balanced diet. But vitamins are just that, supplements. It is important to remember that the human body absorbs vitamins from food more readily than from pills. In addition, science is rapidly discovering dozens of health-supportive phytonutrients in food that work with vitamins to promote health—and these phytonutrients are unavailable in pill form.

Another important point to remember when it comes to vitamins is that you can have too much of a good thing. While large amounts of some vitamins are helpful in specific situations, too much may cause side effects that range from the merely annoying (such as dry skin or sleep disturbances) to the truly dangerous (such as liver damage).

HOW TO TAKE VITAMIN SUPPLEMENTS

• Take vitamin supplements with food to increase absorption. Fat-soluble vitamins should be eaten with food containing some fat.

• If you experience nausea within a half-hour after taking a vitamin, you may not have had enough food in your stomach.

• High doses of vitamins should not be taken at one time. For most efficient absorption, space dosages throughout the day.

WHAT IS VITAMIN D?

Vitamin D may not be one of the most talked-about vitamins in America, but that doesn't mean it isn't among the most important. It helps the body absorb and utilize calcium, making the vitamin essential for the development of bones and teeth. It is in this capacity that vitamin D helps prevent two calcium-deficiency diseases: osteoporosis and rickets (a disease that results in bowlegs and knock-knees). Vitamin D promotes nerve function, protects against muscle weakness, fosters normal muscle contractions, and helps regulate the heartbeat. The vitamin also enhances immune-system function by prompting the thymus gland to create immune-system cells, which in turn destroy bacteria, viruses, and other illness-causing microbes.

Despite its wide-ranging importance, vitamin D is a relatively recent discovery. In 1920, a scientist named Sir Edward Mellanby found that dogs raised exclusively indoors on a limited diet developed the bone disease called rickets. After experimentation, Mellanby found that housebound dogs who regularly consumed cod liver oil (which is rich in vitamin D) didn't develop the condition.

In the early 1930s, researchers isolated in cod liver oil the substance that would later be named vitamin D. Almost simultaneously, researchers discovered that when dehydrocholesterol (a type of cholesterol found in the skin) was irradiated with ultraviolet (UV) light, an identical substance was produced. Because vitamin D could be made by the body when exposed to sunlight, it was nicknamed "the sunshine vitamin." Interestingly, although vitamin D acts like a vitamin and is known to the world as a vitamin, it is chemically a steroid—a hormonal steroid, to be exact—that is built from the same 17-carbon, 4-ring structure as other steroids.

After the body ingests vitamin D through food or supplements, or creates it in the skin through sunlight, the vitamin travels to the liver, where it is metabolized for the body to use. What the body does not use at one given time is stored within fat cells. In other words, the body does not excrete "old, unused" vitamin D before it stockpiles new, incoming vitamin D. Because of this, vitamin D levels can get overly high. The current RDA for vitamin D is 400 IU (international units), and many experts suggest not going over 600 IU on a regular basis without consulting a health care provider.

Vitamin D is found in a few plant foods, yet it is in animal products where it most readily occurs, the best sources being dairy products, eggs, and fish. Fortunately for those who don't get enough sunlight or eat enough foods with naturally occurring vitamin D, the vitamin is commonly added to many processed foods, such as breakfast cereals.

RICKETS—WHAT IS IT?

Vitamin D helps the body absorb and utilize calcium. Without calcium, bones can't grow properly. When growing children don't get enough vitamin D to help their bodies utilize calcium, skeletal deformities, such as bowlegs, knock-knees, and projected ribcage, occur. Because humans can generate their own vitamin D, rickets—as this condition is known—is not a worldwide scourge. Before foods were enriched with vitamin D, the disease was most common among both housebound children and children in low-sun, northern latitudes, who didn't consume large amounts of dairy products, eggs, or fish.

RETHINKING MEDICATION

ANTIBIOTICS: ARE THEY ESSENTIAL?

A recent report published in the *Journal of the American Medical Association* stated that even though antibiotics provide little help for colds, upper respiratory tract infections and bronchitis, doctors still prescribe antibiotics for these conditions. Why? In part, because patients expect their doctors to give them some kind of medication, and many physicians find it easier to oblige than take time out to explain how antibiotics do and don't work. Americans are so enamored of antibiotics that doctors write over 12 million antibiotic prescriptions annually. To learn more about the dangers of antibiotic abuse, contact the Centers For Disease Control and Prevention, 404-332-4555.

PENICILLIN BY THE POUND

Since penicillin's debut in 1941, antibiotic production has shot up from 2 million pounds in 1954 to more than 50 million pounds in 1997. Where is all this medication going? Half of the antibiotics produced annually are prescribed for people; the rest are mixed into livestock feed and used as fertilizers for agricultural crops. The downside to this free-flowing penicillin? New, strong, antibiotic-resistant strains of bacteria.

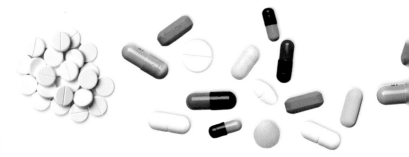

WAIT! BEFORE YOU TAKE THAT PILL . . .
Before asking your doctor for an antibiotic, ask yourself the following questions:

✔ Is my condition caused by bacteria? If not, antibiotics will not work.

✔ Are antibiotics necessary for recovery? If the infection will go away on its own, consider forgoing antibiotics.

✔ Are there alternatives to antibiotics? If herbal or other natural remedies can fight off the infection, consider using one or more of them.

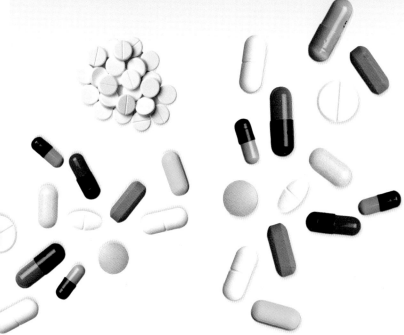

FOOD SOURCES

Food is an important, easily digested source of a wide range of
vitamins. The following are particularly rich in vitamin D:

- Chanterelle mushrooms
- Dandelion greens
- Fatty fish
- Dairy foods
- Egg yolks
- Oatmeal
- Parsley
- Sweet potatoes
- Vitamin D-fortified cereals

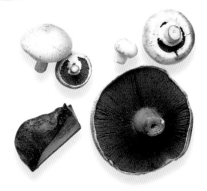

MAKE ROOM

For years, most of the touted sources of vitamin D were animal foods. Of course, there were dandelion greens, oatmeal, parsley, and sweet potatoes. But for the most part, if you wanted to get vitamin D from food, you had to eat fish, eggs, or dairy products. This presented a problem for vegans, who eat no fish, dairy, or eggs. It was even more of a problem for vegans living in sun-deprived climates, who couldn't just step outside for a few minutes and recharge their body's vitamin D stores. Fortunately for everyone— vegan and otherwise—another plant food option was discovered: chanterelle mushrooms. Researchers in Helsinki, Finland, invited 27 women in their mid-20s to lunch every day for three weeks. Nine were served two ounces of ground chanterelle mushrooms, which contained about 560 IU of vitamin D. Nine women received an equivalent amount of vitamin D from a supplement, while the final nine women served as the control group and received no extra vitamin D. During the trial, body levels of vitamin D rose significantly in both the mushroom and supplemented groups, but not in the control group.

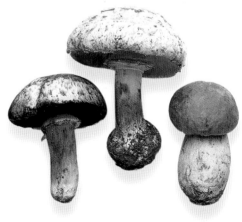

SPECIAL NEEDS

While a daily dose of 400 IU of vitamin D is recommended, the use of the following substances increases the amount of vitamin D needed:

• Alcohol (interferes with the body's metabolism of vitamin D)

• Antacids (can interfere with the body's absorption of vitamin D)

• Barbiturate drugs (increase the body's need for vitamin D)

• Cholesterol-lowering drugs (can decrease the body's vitamin D absorption)

• Corticosteroids (increase the body's need for vitamin D)

CAUTIONS
Vitamin D is considered safe in moderate doses. The following individuals, however, should consult their physicians before ingesting more than 400 to 600 IU of the vitamin a day:

• Individuals with gout. Vitamin D may increase the calcium around damaged joints.

• Rheumatoid arthritis sufferers. Vitamin D may increase the calcium around damaged joints.

• Individuals with hyperthyroidism. Amounts over 400 IU have been found to stimulate the thyroid gland.

VITAMIN D DEFICIENCY

SYMPTOMS OF VITAMIN D-DEFICIENCY

- Anemia
- Bone pain
- Burning sensation in mouth and throat
- Diarrhea
- Insomnia
- Joint pain
- Muscle pain
- Muscle twitching
- Nervousness
- Visual problems

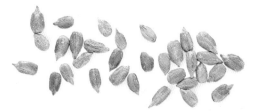

TOO MUCH OF A GOOD THING

Although it is fat-soluble, vitamin D is considered nontoxic because it is not harmful except in extremely high doses. However, excessive vitamin D supplementation may cause the following symptoms in some individuals:

- Appetite loss
- Dizziness
- Excessive thirst
- Headaches
- Kidney damage
- Liver damage
- Nausea

CONDITIONS AND DOSES

ARRHYTHMIA

❒ **Symptoms:** A heartbeat is the sound (heard through a stethoscope) or the vibration (felt when placing a hand on the chest) of the heart as it pumps blood. Like a drummer in a band, the heart keeps a steady pace, which may speed up or slow down as warranted—60 to 80 beats per minute during rest and up to 200 beats per minute during physical exertion. When the heart regularly "misses a beat," the condition is called arrhythmia. The condition can be caused by a diet too high in caffeine, by prescription drugs and smoking, or by an unknown factor. Many people with arrhythmia have no symptoms, while others experience chest discomfort, palpitations, shortness of breath, and/or spells of light-headedness. While the condition is usually harmless, it can be dangerous enough to cause all blood pumping to cease. Thus, if you suspect you have an irregular heartbeat, it is important to consult your physician.

❒ **How Vitamin D Can Help:** Vitamin D helps the heart maintain its regular beating in three ways: The vitamin is involved in the regulation of the heartbeat; it is needed for muscle functioning (the heart is the body's busiest muscle); and vitamin D helps the body effectively absorb and use calcium, a mineral that is also essential for regular cardiac functioning.

❐ **Dosages:** Take 50 to 150 IU of vitamin D three times daily with meals. In addition, get ten minutes of sunlight a day and/or consume daily servings of chanterelle mushrooms, dandelion greens, fatty fish, dairy foods, egg yolks, oatmeal, sweet potatoes, and cereals fortified with vitamin D.

HERE COMES THE SUN

Unlike many vitamins, vitamin D is manufactured in the body. However, to make the vitamin, the body needs sunlight. Simplified, here's how the process works: When the sun's UV rays hit the skin, a cholesterol compound in the skin transforms into vitamin D. About ten minutes of unprotected (meaning without sunscreen) sunshine allows the body to manufacture the RDA of vitamin D: 400 IU. Yet for people at risk for skin cancer, even a short bit of exposure to the sun's UV rays can be dangerous. For them, research has found that food sources and supplements offer the safest way to meet daily requirements for vitamin D.

One of the best-known studies was done by researchers at the National Institutes of Health in Bethesda, MD. For six years scientists studied a group of individuals who took extreme measures to avoid sunlight at all times. This included going outdoors after sundown, keeping windows closed and curtains drawn, and wearing protective clothing. Despite these individuals' near-sunless lifestyle, their vitamin D levels were in the normal range, thanks to a diet rich in D-fortified milk and breakfast cereals.

CONDITIONS AND DOSES

CAVITIES

❐ **Symptoms:** A cavity is a weakened spot in the tooth's enamel, caused when bacteria interact with food particles on teeth, creating decay. Cavity signs include a dull pain in the affected tooth when eating or drinking something hot or cold.

❐ **How Vitamin D Can Help:** Vitamin D cannot remedy a cavity; a visit to the dentist is needed to remove the decay and fill the affected area. Nor can the vitamin prevent bacteria from reacting to food particles and creating decay. What vitamin D can do is strengthen tooth enamel, hardening it and making it more resistant to decay.

❐ **Dosages:** Take 50 to 150 IU of vitamin D three times daily with meals. In addition, get ten minutes of sunlight a day and/or consume daily servings of chanterelle mushrooms, dandelion greens, fatty fish, dairy foods, egg yolks, oatmeal, sweet potatoes, and cereals fortified with vitamin D.

CAVITY FACTS

• Chewable vitamin C tablets can erode tooth enamel and contribute to cavities.

• Avoid carbonated soft drinks, which are high in phosphorus. Many researchers believe that phosphorus promotes loss of calcium from tooth enamel.

• Overly aggressive brushing with a stiff toothbrush can wear away enamel, promoting cavities.

• Individuals eating high-sugar diets experience more cavities. Why? Bacteria in the mouth use sugar to produce an especially strong acid that causes tooth decay.

• According to evidence at archaeological digs, early humans rarely had cavities. Researchers believe their whole-foods, low-sugar diet was the reason why.

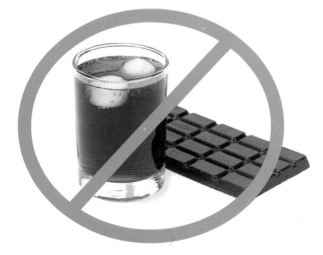

CONDITIONS AND DOSES

FRACTURES

❏ **Symptoms:** Known popularly as a broken bone, a fracture is a common injury. All it takes for a fracture to occur is some type of strong, physical force exerted on one of the body's bones—perhaps the jar of a fall or getting struck with a blunt object. Directly after the break, there may be swelling or bruising in the skin directly over the affected bone, deformity of the area, localized pain that intensifies when the affected area is moved or pressure put on it, and loss of function in the affected area. There may even be a piece of bone that has broken through surrounding tissues and is protruding from the skin.

❏ **How Vitamin D Can Help:** Vitamin D helps build healthy bone cells, making it a necessary nutrient for bone repair. The vitamin also helps the body absorb calcium, a mineral that is necessary for bone regeneration.

❏ **Dosages:** Take 50 to 150 IU of vitamin D three times daily with meals. In addition, get ten minutes of sunlight a day and/or consume chanterelle mushrooms, dandelion greens, fatty fish, dairy foods, egg yolks, oatmeal, sweet potatoes, and cereals fortified with vitamin D.

WHAT KIND IS IT?

Fractures are classified into one or more divisions according to what the actual break looks like. Here are several categories:

• **Compound.** A fracture in which a piece of broken bone has torn through surrounding tissues and is protruding from the skin.
• **Simple or Complete.** A neat snap across the bone, in which the affected bone is snapped into two parts.
• **Incomplete.** The break is limited to a simple crack and the bone has not separated into two parts.
• **Hairline or Stress.** A very small, incomplete fracture.
• **Greenstick.** An incomplete fracture that occurs in young, flexible bones. Instead of snapping horizontally, the bone fractures into a vertical crack.
• **Transverse.** A complete fracture that crosses two or more parallel bones.
• **Oblique.** A diagonal break that travels across one or more parallel bones.
• **Comminuted.** A situation where a segment of bone is shattered into many pieces.
• **Impacted.** One fragment of bone is imbedded into another fragment of bone.

CONDITIONS AND DOSES

LOWER BACK PAIN

❏ **Symptoms:** While backaches are rarely serious, they often are so painful that an individual is immobilized, even hospitalized. This pain—either sudden or chronic—is usually due to pulled, strained or weak back muscles. Causes of backaches include bending at the waist while lifting heavy objects, carrying a heavy handbag, constipation, improper footwear, poor posture, sleeping on a soft mattress, and weak stomach muscles, all of which strain the muscles of the lower back.

❏ **How Vitamin D Can Help:** Vitamin D helps back pain by keeping muscle tissue strong and supple. It also enhances the body's absorption of calcium, a mineral that eases back aches by relaxing cramped muscles.

❏ **Dosages:** Take 50 to 150 IU of vitamin D three times daily with meals. In addition, get ten minutes of sunlight a day and/or consume chanterelle mushrooms, dandelion greens, fatty fish, dairy foods, egg yolks, oatmeal, sweet potatoes, and cereals fortified with vitamin D.

BACK FACTS

- An estimated 80 percent of all Americans are afflicted with back pain at least once in their lives.

- Back pain is one of the most common reasons for hospitalization in the United States.

- Lumbago is the folk term for lower back pain.

- The leading cause of back pain is muscle strain.

- Lower back pain is often chronic, meaning it comes and goes for an extended period of time.

- While x-rays are a routine part of back pain diagnosis, they cannot expose back pain caused by muscle strain.

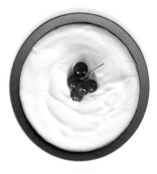

CONDITIONS AND DOSES

LUPUS

❏ **Symptoms:** Lupus is a connective tissue disease. Known in medical-speak as systemic lupus erythematosus, it is a chronic condition in which the body's immune system attacks its own connective tissue cells. While it is not known exactly why some people get lupus, the majority of sufferers are female with a family history of the disease. Furthermore, some researchers link the disease to environmental, hormonal, or viral, factors. Symptoms can range from mild to severe and include fatigue, intermittent, joint pain and swelling, hair loss, intermittent redness around the affected joint, localized chest pain that may be accompanied by coughing, morning stiffness, photosensitivity, and rashes (especially across the nose and cheeks). In some individuals with lupus, the immune system eventually attacks kidney cells, leading to kidney disease.

❏ **How Vitamin D Can Help:** Vitamin D cannot cure or even prevent lupus. What it can do is help protect bones. This is particularly important for people who take glucocorticoid medications (such as prednisone) to control lupus, since these medications frequently cause bone loss.

❏ **Dosages:** Take 50 to 150 IU of vitamin D three times daily with meals. In addition consume chanterelle mushrooms, dandelion greens, fatty fish, dairy foods, egg yolks, oatmeal, sweet potatoes, and cereals fortified with vitamin D.

LUPUS FACTS

• The word "lupus" means "wolf' in Latin. The disease's name refers to the rash that falls across the nose and cheeks, giving Lupus sufferers a wolf-like appearance.

• Nine to ten time as many women as men have lupus.

• Women of Asian descent are more likely to get lupus than women of African, European or Native American descent.

• Lupus often occurs for the first time during pregnancy.

• Lupus usually occurs between the ages of 15 and 30.

• Autoimmune diseases, such as lupus, leave sufferers with increased susceptibility to viral illnesses, such as colds and flus.

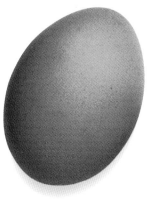

CONDITIONS AND DOSES

MYELOGENOUS LEUKEMIA

❐ **Symptoms:** Myelogenous leukemia is also called myeloid, myelocytic, chronic myelogenous, or granulocytic leukemia. It is characterized by an overproduction of a cancerous version of white blood cells called granulocytes that are formed in the bone marrow. While it is not known what causes the disorder, it occurs most often in individuals between the ages of 35 and 60. In up to a third of the cases, individuals have the disease for two to five years before symptoms occur, and they discover they have the disease only when a routine blood test shows abnormal results. Signs can include bone pain, bruising, increased susceptibility to infectious illnesses, pressure under the left ribs caused by an enlarged spleen, swollen lymph nodes, unexplained fevers, and unexplained weight loss. The disease is a progressive one, meaning it grows continuously worse with time.

❐ **How Vitamin D Can Help:** Currently, conventional treatment for myelogenous leukemia is high-dose chemotherapy with total-body irradiation, followed by bone marrow transplantation. Vitamin D has been shown to be beneficial after bone marrow transplantation, helping the body generate healthy new blood cells and bone cells.

❒ **Dosages:** Before taking any supplement, please consult your physician. With your doctor's go-ahead, take 50 to 150 IU of vitamin D three times daily with meals. In addition, get ten minutes of sunlight a day and/or consume daily servings of chanterelle mushrooms, dandelion greens, fatty fish, dairy foods, egg yolks, oatmeal, sweet potatoes, and cereals fortified with vitamin D.

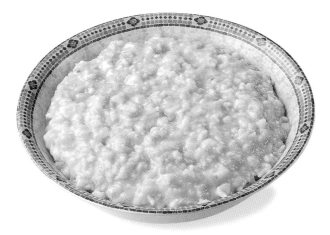

CONDITIONS AND DOSES

OSTEOARTHRITIS

❐ **Symptoms:** Osteoarthritis, also known simply as arthritis, is one of the most common disorders known to humans, affecting up to 80 percent of all individuals over the age of 60. Caused by simple wear and tear of a joint, arthritis is considered a degenerative disease. Symptoms include mild to moderately severe pain in a joint during or after use, discomfort in a joint during a weather change, swelling in an affected joint, and loss of flexibility in a joint.

❐ **How Vitamin D Can Help:** Several studies have shown that individuals with low levels of vitamin D are up to three times more likely to get arthritis than individuals who get at least 200 IU of vitamin D a day. Vitamin D helps build healthy bones and cartilage, thus acting both to prevent osteoarthritis and slow the progression of the disease.

❐ **Dosages:** Take 50 to 150 IU of vitamin D three times daily with meals. In addition, get ten minutes of sunlight a day and/or consume daily servings of chanterelle mushrooms, dandelion greens, fatty fish, dairy foods, egg yolks, oatmeal, sweet potatoes, cereals fortified with vitamin D.

VITAMIN D SLOWS ARTHRITIS
Individuals who suffer from arthritis may be able to slow the disease's progression with daily doses of vitamin D. Researchers at Boston University Medical Center examined the knees of 556 patients during a two-year period. The findings? Patients who showed the most progressive arthritic knee damage were those exhibiting the lowest levels of vitamin D. The body needs vitamin D to repair the damage that arthritis causes in both bones and cartilage.

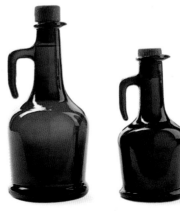

CONDITIONS AND DOSES

OSTEOPOROSIS

❐ **Symptoms:** We tend to think of bones as made up of inert matter. The truth is, however, that bones are comprised of living, changing tissues, that produce blood cells and act as a storehouse for calcium and phosphate. Should the calcium stores within bones become depleted, the resulting condition is called osteoporosis. The term osteoporosis comes from the Greek words *osteon* ("bone") and *porus* ("pore" or "passage"), and the disease is marked by increasing porosity in the bones. As bones become more porous, they grow fragile and are easily broken. In addition to fractures (especially of the hips, vertebrae, and wrists), individuals with osteoporosis often suffer from lower back pain and from moderate to severe stooped posture as bones are unable to support the body's full weight. While men do get osteoporosis, they don't get it as often as women do, thanks to their heavy, calcium-dense bones. Women—especially those with light skeletal frames—have less calcium to begin with, which increases their susceptibility to the disease. Other risk factors include low calcium and vitamin D intake, a sedentary lifestyle, and corticosteroid use.

❐ **How Vitamin D Can Help:** American and European research has found that 40 percent of elderly men and women with osteoporosis-caused hip fractures have a vitamin D deficientcy. Other studies have shown that supplementing postmenopausal women with vitamin D increases their bone density. How does vitamin D do all this? The nutrient is essential for building new bone tissue. It also helps the body absorb calcium, a mineral that keeps bones strong and dense.

❏ **Dosages:** Take 50 to 150 IU of vitamin D three times daily with meals. In addition, get ten minutes of sunlight a day and/or consume daily servings of chanterelle mushrooms, dandelion greens, fatty fish, dairy foods, egg yolks, oatmeal, sweet potatoes, and cereals fortified with vitamin D.

VITAMIN D: A TEAM PLAYER
Vitamin D works with calcium to build bone mass. Just how much mass this nutritional team can build was looked at by researchers at the USDA Human Nutrition Research Center on Aging at Tufts University in Boston. The study followed 176 men and 213 women aged 65 and older. Every day for three years, test subjects took either 500 mg of calcium plus 700 IU of vitamin D, or a placebo. After one year, the supplement-taking group had significantly greater overall bone density than the placebo group. In the second and third years, the improvement in the supplement group's bone density was so great that their risk of fracture was cut in half. The placebo group actually lost overall bone mass.

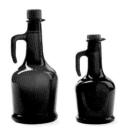

CONDITIONS AND DOSES

PSORIASIS

❏ **Symptoms:** Normal skin cells mature and pass from the dermis to the epidermis in about 28 days. When psoriasis is present, skin cells make the same trip in eight days, causing noncontagious patches of silvery or red scaly areas, patches that often spread to cover larger and larger areas. Skin cells generally fluctuate between this "accelerated growth" and remission, when they grow normally. Although psoriasis is often hereditary, it isn't yet known exactly what causes it: Faulty utilization of fats, poor liver function, depressed immune system, and build up of unhealthy toxins in the colon have all been linked to the disease.

❏ **How Vitamin D Can Help:** When applied topically as Activated Vitamin D_3 Ointment (also called Dovonex), vitamin D helps stop psoriasis symptoms by slowing accelerated skin cell growth. Vitamin D is considered a steroid hormone, that behaves similarly to cortisone, another steroid hormone which is also prescribed to slow accelerated psoriasis skin cell growth. The other common psoriasis treatment is ultraviolet (UV) therapy. While it was believed that the UVA and UVB rays in sunlight were responsible for reducing psoriasis symptoms, some researchers now believe it is actually the increased vitamin D created by the body when exposed to UV light that is responsible for slowing these symptoms.

❒ **Dosages:** Take 50 to 150 IU of vitamin D three times daily with meals. In addition, get ten minutes of sunlight a day and/or consume daily servings of chanterelle mushrooms, dandelion greens, fatty fish, dairy foods, egg yolks, oatmeal, sweet potatoes, and cereals fortified with vitamin D.

A NATURAL PROTECTOR
Looking for an easy way to protect your bones? Something natural that you can do everyday to prevent getting osteoporosis in the future? Look no further than vitamin D. Finnish researchers gave 341 elderly people (mostly women aged 75 and older), annual large-dose injections of vitamin D over a five-year period. The results? These individuals experienced far fewer bone fractures than the 458 people in a control group who did not receive the vitamin.

CONDITIONS AND DOSES

RHEUMATOID ARTHRITIS

❐ **Symptoms:** Rheumatoid arthritis is an autoimmune disease in which the body's immune system attacks itself. Though the ailment is not well-understood, it is believed that an unidentified virus stimulates the body to attack its own joints. Symptoms include pain and swelling in the smaller joints of hands and feet, overall aching and/or stiffness after periods of motionlessness, local fever in affecting joints.

❐ **How Vitamin D Can Help:** Whether from supplements or food sources, vitamin D can help protect bones. This is particularly important for people with rheumatoid arthritis who take glucocorticoid medications (such as prednisone), because these medications can cause bone loss.

❐ **Dosages:** Take 50 to 150 IU of vitamin D three times daily with meals. In addition, get ten minutes of sunlight a day and/or consume chanterelle mushrooms, dandelion greens, fatty fish, dairy foods, egg yolks, oatmeal, sweet potatoes, and cereals fortified with vitamin D.

RHEUMATOID FACTS

• Currently 2.1 million Americans have rheumatoid arthritis.

• Two-thirds of rheumatoid arthritis sufferers are women.

• The majority of rheumatoid arthritis sufferers are under age 40.

• Rheumatoid arthritis' typical age of onset is between 25 and 50 years old.

• Unlike osteoarthritis, which is characterized by a popping or clicking noise in the joints, rheumatoid arthritis is marked by joint noises that sound like crinkling cellophane.

• Lyme disease can be mistaken for rheumatoid arthritis, causing many of the same symptoms.

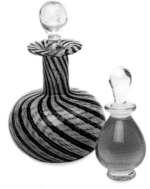

CONDITIONS AND DOSES

SEASONAL AFFECTIVE DISORDER

❐ **Symptoms:** Seasonal Affective Disorder (SAD) is a type of depression caused by the lack of sunlight that occurs in late fall, winter, and/or early spring. Scientists believe the lack of light triggers biochemical changes in the brain. Symptoms occur only during a specific time frame, usually late fall to early spring. They include anxiety, carbohydrate cravings, crying spells, decreased energy level, decreased libido, lethargy, low-grade headaches, impaired concentration, increase in sleep, irritability, malaise, and weight gain.

❐ **How Vitamin D Can Help:** Light therapy is the most traditional treatment for SAD. Promising new research, however, shows that supplements of vitamin D—a vitamin made by the body when exposed to sunlight—are just as effective as actual ultraviolet (UV) light in regulating the brain chemicals responsible for depression. Note: If you suspect you have SAD, consult a physician.

❐ **Dosages:** Take 50 to 150 IU of vitamin D three times daily with meals. In addition, get ten minutes of sunlight a day and/or consume daily servings of chanterelle mushrooms, dandelion greens, fatty fish, dairy foods, egg yolks, oatmeal, sweet potatoes, and cereals fortified with vitamin D.

MOOD BUSTER

For individuals who suffer from Seasonal Affective Disorder (SAD), the lack of sunlight in late fall and early winter is enough to send them into a several-month slump. Luckily for those who can't get away to a sun-drenched island getaway, there's vitamin D. In a recent study, college students who took 400 IU of vitamin D daily during the winter reported feeling more enthusiastic, inspired, and alert than those who took a placebo.

CONDITIONS AND DOSES

SPRAINED MUSCLES

❑ **Symptoms:** A sprain occurs when a violent twist or stretch causes the joint to move outside its normal range of movement, injuring the muscles and/or ligaments that connect the bones. The result is rapid swelling in the injured area, impaired joint function, pain and tenderness.

❑ **How Vitamin D Can Help:** Vitamin D helps sprained muscles by helping to repair damaged tissue and generate healthy new tissue. It also enhances the body's absorption of calcium, a mineral needed for connective tissue repair.

❑ **Dosages:** Take 50 to 150 IU of vitamin D three times daily with meals. In addition, get ten minutes of sunlight a day and/or consume chanterelle mushrooms, dandelion greens, fatty fish, dairy foods, egg yolks, oatmeal, sweet potatoes, and cereals fortified with vitamin D.

SPRAIN FACTS

• The most frequently-sprained areas are the ankle, back, fingers, knee, and wrist.

• Most sprains are able to bear weight within 24 hours and area fully healed within two weeks.

• Sprains can be prevented by stretching muscles before and after physical activity.

• Immediately after spraining a muscle, apply ice or cold packs to the injured area for the first 24 hours to reduce inflammation.

• If possible, elevate the affected area and use a compression wrap (such as an Ace bandage) to reduce and prevent swelling.

• Repeated minor sprains in one area—such as the ankle— can lead to weakening of the affected joint.

• Once the sprain has healed, taping, bracing or wrapping the affected joint before physical activity can reduce the chances of re-injuring the area.

CONDITIONS AND DOSES

SUSCEPTIBILITY TO INFECTIOUS ILLNESSES

❏ **Symptoms:** The average American gets two or three colds and one bout of flu each year. If you suffer from more than this, there's a chance you may have a poorly functioning immune system—which increases your susceptibility to infectious illnesses. Some people are born with weak immune systems, while others undermine their immunity with heavy drinking, poor diet, recreational drug use, smoking, or chronic stress.

❏ **How Vitamin D Can Help:** While vitamin D is most often thought of as a bone-builder, it also plays a role in maintaining immunity. The vitamin works by prompting the thymus gland to create immune-system cells, which in turn destroy bacteria, viruses, and other illness-causing microbes.

❏ **Dosages:** Take 50 to 150 IU of vitamin D three times daily with meals. In addition, get ten minutes of sunlight a day and/or consume daily servings of chanterelle mushrooms, dandelion greens, fatty fish, dairy foods, egg yolks, oatmeal, sweet potatoes, and cereals fortified with vitamin D.

A "NEW" IMMUNE BOOSTER

Think about the nutrients that help build a healthy immune system and chances are vitamins like A, C, and E jump to mind. And with good reason—all are important antioxidants and immune-system helpers. But what about vitamin D? Yes, you read it right. The "sunshine vitamin" is developing quite a reputation these days as a key immune-system player. In fact, when researchers at the University of Wisconsin Madison tested lab animals deficient in vitamin D, they found that the thymus gland was not doing its job—which is generating a sufficient number of immune-system cells. Furthermore, it took two months of a diet with normal daily vitamin D levels to restore proper immunity.

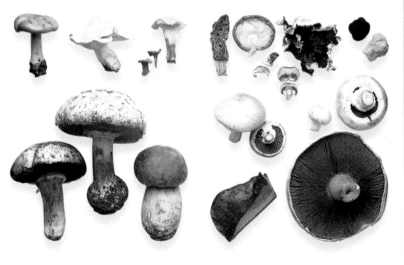

VITAMIN D COMPANION

VITAMIN D: A COMPANION TREATMENT

Good news for arthritis sufferers: Vitamin D is helpful when used with drug therapy, according to a recent study of individuals taking 5.6 mg of prednisone daily. In addition to prednisone, test subjects took 1,000 mg of calcium carbonate daily and 500 IU of vitamin D daily. After two years, individuals using these nutritional supplements gained bone mass, while a group taking placebo pills actually lost bone mass.

SAFETY CHECKLIST
Before taking any vitamin, ask yourself the following
questions:

• Have I done any background research on the vitamin?

• What condition am I taking this vitamin for?

• Am I taking other medications, herbs, or nutrients that may
affect the vitamin's functioning?

• Do I have any pre existing condition that is contraindicated?

• Am I pregnant, trying to conceive, or nursing?

• Have I spoken to my physician, a naturopathic doctor, or a
nutritionist before taking the vitamin?

• Do I know the proper dosages for the vitamin?

ALTERNATIVE HEALTH STRATEGIES

Herbs, vitamins, minerals—of course these contribute to good health. But creating general well-being involves more than simply taking supplements. Good health has to do with various quality-of-life issues that can aggravate or cause stress, thus harming health. Here are some additional ways to help keep yourself well.

Improve Your Eating Habits
Here are the five main eating strategies people follow; consider finding the most healthful one that works with your lifestyle.

- OMNIVOROUS
- PISCATORIAL
- MACROBIOTIC
- VEGAN
- VEGETARIAN

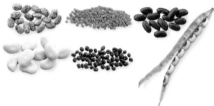

Get More Exercise
Whether it's walking or weightlifting, exercise can help you feel better. Try any of these types:

- STRETCHING
- AEROBICS
- STRENGTH TRAINING

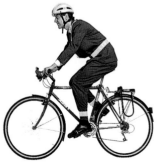

Simple Ways To Ease Stress

In addition to exercise and healthful eating, here are some more techniques—old and new—for easing stress and increasing relaxation.

- GET ENOUGH SLEEP
- MEDITATE REGULARLY
- GIVE UP JUNK FOOD
- ADOPT A PET
- SURROUND YOURSELF WITH SUPPORTIVE PEOPLE
- LIMIT YOUR EXPOSURE TO CHEMICALS
- TAKE YOUR VITAMINS
- ENJOY YOURSELF

ONE-MINUTE STRESS REDUCER

Stress is one of the top health hazards we face today. Unfortunately, it's impossible to go through life without the irritations that make us tense. Fortunately, there *is* something you can do to minimize their power to aggravate you. It's called deep breathing, and it can be done anywhere and anytime you need to calm and center yourself. Here's how to do it:

1. Inhale deeply through your nose.
2. Hold your breath for up to three seconds, then exhale through your mouth.
3. Continue as needed.

Deep breathing pulls a person's attention away from a given stressor and refocuses it on his or her breath. This type of breathing is not only comforting (thanks to its rhythmic quality), but also has been shown to lower rapid pulse and shallow respiration—two temporary symptoms of stress.

GET MOVING

Ask medical experts to name one stay-young strategy and there's a good chance "exercise" will be the answer. And with good reason. Exercise, whether a gentle walk around the block or a full-tilt weight-lifting session, strengthens the heart, lowers the body's resting heart rate, builds muscles, boosts circulation to the body and the brain, revs up the metabolism, and burns calories. All of which can keep a person looking and feeling his or her best. To be effective, exercise must be performed several times a week. Aim for at least three sessions. However, there's more than one kind of exercise. For optimum health, try a combination of aerobic exercise and strength training. And don't forget to stretch before and after each workout!

STRETCHING

❒ **What It Is:** Any movement that stretches muscles. Examples include bending at the waist and touching the toes, sitting with legs outstretched in front of you, and rolling your neck. Stretch for eight to twelve minutes before every workout and again after you exercise.

❒ **Why It's Important:** Muscles act like springs. If a muscle is short and tight, it loses the ability to absorb shock. The less shock a muscle can absorb, the more strain there is on the joints. Thus, stretching maintains flexibility, which in turn prevents injuries. Because we often lose our regular range of motion with age, stretching is especially important for older adults to prevent sprains, strains and falls.

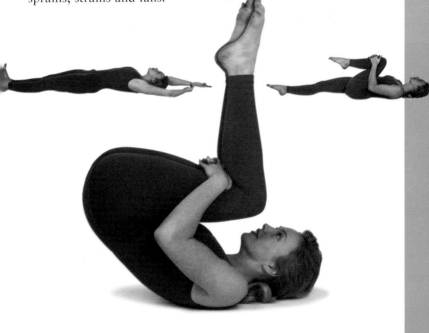

GET MOVING

AEROBICS

❑ **What It Is:** Any activity that uses large muscle groups, is maintained continuously for 15 minutes or more, and is rhythmic in nature. Examples include aerobic dance, jogging, skating, and walking. Ideally, you should aim for three to six aerobic workouts per week.

❑ **Why It's Important:** Aerobic exercise trains the heart, lungs, and cardiovascular system to process and deliver oxygen more quickly and efficiently to every part of the body. As the heart muscle becomes stronger and more efficient, a larger amount of blood can be pumped with each stroke. Fewer strokes are then required to rapidly transport oxygen to all parts of the body.

STRENGTH TRAINING

❒ **What It Is:** Any activity that improves the condition of your muscles by making repeated movements against a force. Examples include lifting large or small weights, sit-ups, stair-stepping, and isometrics.

❒ **Why It's Important:** Strength training makes it easier to move heavy loads, whether they require carrying, pushing, pulling or lifting, as well as to participate in sports that require strength. The exercises are of various kinds. Some require changing the length of the muscle while maintaining the level of tension, others involve using special equipment to vary the tension in the muscles, and some entail contracting a muscle while maintaining its length.

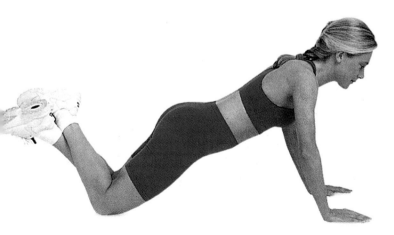

EATING SMART

A balanced diet is the foundation of good health. For proof, just read the numerous medical studies that link healthful eating with disease prevention and disease reversal. These same studies connect high fat intake, high sodium consumption, and diets with too much protein to numerous illnesses, including cancer, cardiovascular diseases, diverticular diseases, hypertension, and heart disease. But what exactly is a balanced diet? Generally speaking, it is a diet comprised of carbohydrates, dietary fiber, fat, protein, water, 13 vitamins, and 20 minerals. More specifically, it is a diet built around a wide variety of fruits, legumes, whole grains, and vegetables. Alcohol, animal protein, high-fat foods, high-sodium foods, highly-sugared foods, sodas, and processed foods are consumed sparingly, if at all.

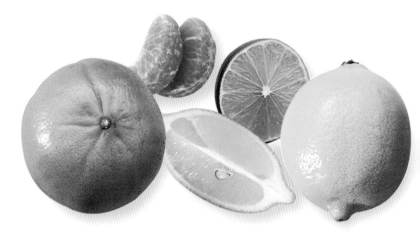

OMNIVOROUS

❏ **On the Menu:** Plant-based foods, dairy products, eggs, fish, seafood, red meats, organ meats, poultry.

❏ **Foods That Are Avoided:** None. Everything is fair game.

❏ **How Healthy Is It?** It depends. Someone who eats eggs, poultry or meat every day, chooses refined snacks over whole foods, and gets only one or two daily servings of fruits and vegetables will not be as healthy as a person who limits meat (the general dietary term for any "flesh foods," including poultry and fish) to two or three times a week, chooses water over soft drinks, and gets the recommended five or more daily servings of fruits and vegetables. Complaints about traditional omnivorous diets revolve around the diet's high level of cholesterol and saturated fat (found in animal-based foods), which increases one's risk of cancer, diabetes, heart disease, and obesity. However, an omnivorous diet can be a healthful one, provided thoughtful choices are made. To keep cholesterol and saturated fat to a minimum and nutrients to a maximum, eat five or more daily servings of fruits and vegetables, choose whole grains over refined grains, enjoy daily legume or soyfood protein sources, and limit the use of animal foods.

EATING SMART

MACROBIOTIC

❏ **On the Menu:** Plant-based foods, fish, very limited amounts of salt.

❏ **Foods That Are Avoided:** Dairy products, eggs, foods with artificial ingredients, hot spices, mass-produced foods, organ meats, peppers, potatoes, poultry, red meats, shellfish, warm drinks, refined foods.

❏ **How Healthy Is It?** Macrobiotics is based on a system created inn the early 1900s by Japanese philosopher George Ohsawa. The diet consists of 50 percent whole grains, 20 to 30 percent vegetables, and 5 to 10 percent beans, sea vegetables, and soy foods. The remainder of the diet is composed of white-meat fish, fruits, and nuts. The diet's low amounts of saturated fat, absence of processed foods, and emphasis on high-fiber foods, such as whole grains and vegetables, may promote cardiovascular health. Because soy and sea vegetables contain cancer-fighting compounds, macrobiotics is often recommended to help treat cancer. However, critics worry that the diet's limited variety of food can leave followers lacking in certain vitamins and important cancer-fighting phytonutrients.

PISCATORIAL

❒ **On the Menu:** Plant-based foods, dairy products, eggs, fish, seafood.

❒ **Foods That Are Avoided:** Red meats, organ meats, poultry.

❒ **How Healthy Is It?** Like an omnivorous diet, a piscatorial diet is as healthy as a person makes it. Individuals who eat high-fat and highly processed foods, fail to get the recommended daily number of vegetables and fruits, and eschew whole grains for processed grains will not enjoy optimum health. That said, individuals who are conscientious about eating a balanced, varied diet, and who limit fish and seafood intake to two or three times per week, can expect a lower risk of heart disease. Since many oily fish contain omega-3 fatty acids, eating oily fish in moderation has been found to help lower blood cholesterol. Be aware, however, that oily saltwater fish, such as shark, swordfish and tuna, have been found to carry mercury in their tissues; many health authorities recommend eating these varieties no more than once or twice a week. Also, due to overfishing, many fish species are now threatened, including bluefin tuna, Pacific perch, Chilean sea bass, Chinook salmon, and swordfish. For additional information on endangered fish, visit the University of Michigan's Endangered Species Update at www.umich.edu/~esuupdate, or the Fish and Wildlife Information Exchange at http://fwie.fe.vt.edu.

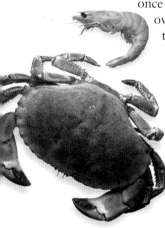

EATING SMART

VEGAN

❏ **On the Menu:** Plant-based foods.

❏ **Foods That Are Avoided:** Dairy, eggs, fish, seafood, red meats, organ meats, poultry. Also avoided are foods made by animals or processed with animal parts, such as gelatin, honey, marshmallows made with animal gelatin, white sugar processed with bone char.

❏ **How Healthy Is It?** A vegan (pronounced VEE-gun) diet can be extremely healthy. Like the vegetarian diet, a vegan diet has been shown by numerous studies to lower blood pressure and prevent heart disease. In addition, the high fiber intake cuts one's risk of diverticular disease and colon cancer. Yet because vegans do not eat dairy products or eggs, they must be more conscientious than vegetarians about either eating plant foods with vitamin B_{12} and vitamin D, or taking supplements of these nutrients.

VEGETARIAN

❒ **On the Menu:** Plant-based foods, dairy, eggs.

❒ **Foods That Are Avoided:** Fish, gelatin, seafood, red meats, organ meats, poultry.

❒ **How Healthy Is It?** A vegetarian diet can be very healthy when done right. Fortunately, this isn't hard. Dietary science has debunked theories of "protein combining" popular in the 1960s and 1970s, leaving today's vegetarians to worry only about eating a wide variety of whole foods, including beans, fruits, grains, low-fat dairy products, nuts, soy foods, and vegetables. A varied daily diet insures enough protein, calcium, and other nutrients for vegetarians of all ages, including children, pregnant individuals, and the elderly. A well-chosen vegetarian eating plan has been shown by numerous studies to lower blood pressure, decrease one's risk of breast cancer, and prevent heart disease. In addition, the diet's high fiber levels cut the risk of diverticular disease and colon cancer.

NUTRIENT KNOW-HOW

Vitamins and minerals are known collectively as nutrients. Name a body function, whether carbohydrate metabolism, nerve cell replication, or wound healing, and you'll find one or more of these nutrients at work. The best place to look for vitamins and minerals? In the food you eat every day. Indeed, if you eat a well-balanced diet there's a good chance you'll get all the nutrients your body needs. But if you are ill, pregnant, eat an inadequate diet, drink more than two alcoholic or caffeinated drinks per day,

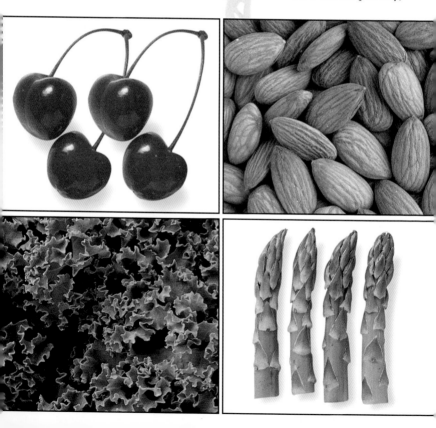

are under stress, are taking certain medications, or have difficulty absorbing certain nutrients, you may need to supplement your diet with one or more vitamins or minerals. Supplements generally come in tablet and capsule form, although some health food stores also carry liquid supplements. Whichever form you choose, doses are measured by weight in milligrams (mg); in micrograms (mcg); or in the universal standard known as international units (IU).

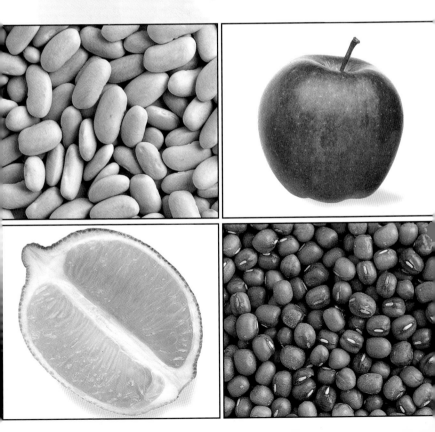

VITAMIN A

(beta carotene, retinol)

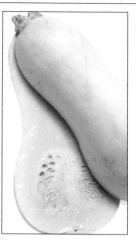

What It Does: Vitamin A is found in two forms: performed vitamin A, known as retinol, and provitamin A, called beta carotene. Retinol is found only in foods of animal origin. Beta carotene, a carotenoid, is a pigment found in plants. Beta carotene has a slight nutritional edge, boasting antioxidant properties and the ability to help lower harmful cholesterol levels. Regardless of the form, vitamin A is essential for good vision; promotes healthy skin, hair, and mucous membranes; stimulates wound healing; and is necessary for proper development of bones and teeth.

Recommended Daily Allowance: Men, 5,000 IU (or 3 mg beta carotene); women, 4,000 IU (or 2.4 mg beta carotene).

Food Sources: Orange and yellow fruits and vegetables, dark green leafy vegetables, whole milk, cream, butter, organ meats.

Toxic Dosage: When taken in excess of 10,000 IU daily, prolonged use of vitamin A supplements can cause abdominal pain, amenorrhea, dry skin, enlarged liver or spleen, hair loss, headaches, itching, joint pain, nausea, vision problems, vomiting.

Enemies: Antibiotics, cholesterol-lowering drugs, heavy laxative use.

Deficiency Symptoms: Because vitamin A is fat-soluble, it is stored in the body's fat for a long time, making deficiency uncommon. However, deficiency symptoms include dryness of the conjunctiva and cornea, frequent colds, insomnia, night blindness, reproductive difficulties, respiratory infections.

VITAMIN B$_1$

(thiamine)

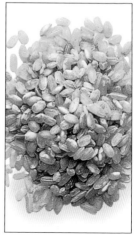

What It Does: Maintains normal nervous system functioning, helps metabolize carbohydrates, proteins, and fats; assists in blood formation and circulation; optimizes cognitive activity and brain function; regulates the body's appetite; protects the body from the degenerative effects of alcohol consumption, environmental pollution, and smoking.

Minimum Recommended Daily Allowance: Men, 1.5 mg; women, 1.1 mg.

Food Sources: Brewer's yeast, broccoli, brown rice, egg yolks, fish, legumes, peanuts, peas, pork, prunes, oatmeal, raisins, rice bran, soybeans, wheat germ, whole grains.

Toxic Dosage: There is no know toxicity level for vitamin B$_1$.

Enemies: Antibiotics, a diet high in simple carbohydrates, heavy physical exertion, oral contraceptives, sulfa drugs.

Deficiency Symptoms: Appetite loss, confusion, fatigue, heart arrhythmia, nausea, mood swings. Severe deficiency can lead to beriberi, a crippling disease characterized by convulsions, diarrhea, edema, gastrointestinal problems, heart failure, mental confusion, nerve damage, paralysis, severe weight loss.

VITAMIN B₂

(riboflavin, vitamin G)
What It Does: Helps metabolize carbohydrates, fats, and proteins; allows skin, nail, and hair tissues to utilize oxygen; aids in red blood cell formation and antibody production; promotes cell respiration; maintains proper nerve function, eyes, and adrenal glands.
Minimum Recommended Daily Allowance: Men, 1.7 mg; women, 1.3 mg; pregnant women, 1.6 mg.
Food Sources: Cheese, egg yolks, fish, legumes, milk, poultry, spinach, whole grains, yogurt.
Toxic Dosage: There is no known toxicity level for this vitamin, although nervousness and rapid heartbeat have been reported with daily dosages of 10 mg.
Enemies: Alcohol, oral contraceptives, strenuous exercise.
Deficiency Symptoms: Cracks at the corners of the mouth, dermatitis, dizziness, hair loss, insomnia, itchy or burning eyes, light sensitivity, mouth sores, impaired thinking, inflammation of the tongue, rashes.

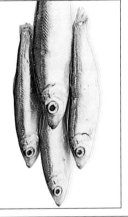

VITAMIN B₅

(pantothenic acid)
What It Does: Helps produce adrenal hormones, antibodies, and various neurotransmitters; reduces skin inflammation; speeds healing of wounds; helps convert food to energy.
Minimum Recommended Daily Allowance: 4 mg.
Food Sources: Beef, eggs, beans, brown rice, lentils, mushrooms, nuts, peas, pork, saltwater fish, sweet potatoes.
Toxic Dosages: There is no known toxicity level for this vitamin; however, doses above 10 mg can cause diarrhea in some individuals.
Deficiency Symptoms: Vitamin B₅ deficiency is extremely rare and is likely to occur only with starvation.

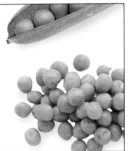

VITAMIN B₆

(pyridoxine)
What It Does: Involved in more bodily functions than nearly any other nutrient. It helps the body metabolize carbohydrates, fats and proteins; supports immune function; helps build red blood cells; assists in transmission of nerve impulses; maintains the body's sodium and potassium balance; helps synthesize RNA and DNA.
Minimum Recommended Daily Allowance: Men, 2 mg; women, 1.6 mg; pregnant women, 2.2 mg.
Food Sources: Avocados, bananas, beans, blackstrap molasses, brown rice, carrots, corn, fish, nuts, sunflower seeds.
Toxic Dosage: Levels of 2,000 to 5,000 mg can cause numbness in the hands and feet, and insomnia.
Deficiency Symptoms: Vitamin B₆ deficiency is rare. Symptoms include depression, fatigue, flaky skin, headaches, insomnia, irritability, muscle weakness, nausea.

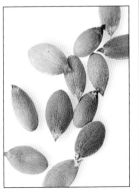

VITAMIN B₁₂

(cobalamin)
What It Does: Regulates formation of red blood cells, helps the body utilize iron; converts carbohydrates, fats, and proteins into energy; aids in cellular formation and cellular longevity; prevents nerve damage; maintains fertility; promotes normal growth.
Minimum Recommended Daily Allowance: Adults, 2 mg; pregnant women, 2.2 mg.
Food Sources: Brewer's yeast, dairy products, eggs, organ meats, seafood, sea vegetables, tempeh.
Toxic Dosage: There is no known toxicity level for vitamin B₁₂.
Enemies: Anticoagulant drugs, anti gout medication, potassium supplements.
Deficiency Symptoms: While deficiency is rare, individuals who do not eat animal products are at risk unless they fortify their diets with plant-sources such as brewer's yeast and sea vegetables. Symptoms include back pain, body odor, constipation, dizziness, fatigue, moodiness, numbness and tingling in the arms and legs, ringing in the ears, muscle weakness, tongue inflammation, weight loss. Severe deficiency can lead to pernicious anemia, characterized by abdominal pain, stiffness in the arms and legs, a tendency to bleed, yellowish cast to the skin, permanent nerve damage, death.

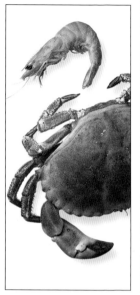

VITAMIN C

(ascorbic acid)
What It Does: Protects against pollution and infection, enhances immunity; aids in growth and repair of both bone and tissue by helping the body produce collagen; maintains adrenal gland function; helps the body absorb iron; aids in production of antistress hormones; reduces cholesterol levels; lowers high blood pressure; prevents artherosclerosis.
Minimum Recommended Daily Allowance: Adults, 60 mg; pregnant women, 70 mg.
Food Sources: Berries, cantaloupe, citrus fruits, broccoli, leafy greens, mangoes, papayas, peppers, persimmons, pineapple, tomatoes.
Toxic Dosage: Doses larger than 10,000 mg can cause diarrhea, stomach irritation, or increased kidney stone formation. **Enemies:** Alcohol, analgesics, antidepressants, anticoagulants, oral contraceptives, smoking, steroids.
Deficiency Symptoms: Bleeding gums, easy bruising, fatigue, reduced resistance to colds and other infections, slow healing of wounds, weight loss. Severe deficiency can lead to scurvy, a sometimes-fatal disease characterized by aching bones, muscle weakness, and swollen and bleeding gums.

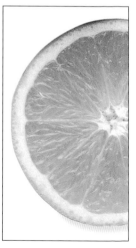

VITAMIN D

(calciferol, ergosterol)

What It Does: Helps the body utilize calcium and phosphorus; promotes normal development of bones and teeth; assists in thyroid function; maintains normal blood clotting; helps regulate heartbeat, nerve function, and muscle contraction.

Minimum Recommended Daily Allowance: Adults, 200 IU (5 mcg); pregnant women, 400 IU (10 mcg).

Food Sources: Dandelion greens, dairy products, eggs, fatty saltwater fish, parsley, sweet potatoes, vegetable oils.

Toxic Dosage: Daily doses higher than 400 IU can lead to raised blood calcium levels and calcium deposits of the heart, liver, and kidney.

Enemies: Antacids, cholesterol-lowering drugs, cortisone drugs.

Deficiency Symptoms: The body naturally manufactures about 200 IU of vitamin D when exposed to ten minutes of ultraviolet light, making deficiency rare. Symptoms include bone weakening, diarrhea, insomnia, muscle twitches, vision disturbances. Severe deficiency can lead to rickets, a disease that results in bone defects such as bowlegs and knock-knees.

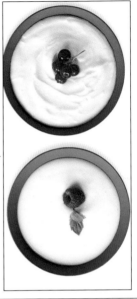

VITAMIN E

(tocopherol)

What It Does: Prevents unstable molecules known as free radicals from damaging cells and tissue; accelerates wound healing; protects lung tissue from inhaled pollutants; aids in functioning of the immune system; endocrine system, and sex glands; improves circulation; promotes normal blood clotting.

Minimum Recommended Daily Allowance: Men, 15 IU (10 mg); women, 12 IU (8 mg); pregnant women, 15 IU (10 mg).

Food Sources: Avocados, dark green leafy vegetables, eggs, legumes, nuts, organ meats, seafood, seeds, soybeans.

Toxic Dosage: Although there is no established toxicity level of vitamin E, the vitamin has blood-thinning properties; individuals who are taking anticoagulant medications or have clotting deficiencies should avoid vitamin E.

Enemies: High temperatures and overcooking reduce vitamin E levels in food.

Deficiency Symptoms: Vitamin E deficiency is rare. Deficiency symptoms include fluid retention, infertility, miscarriage, muscle degeneration.

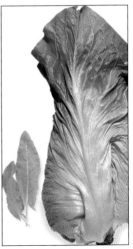

CALCIUM

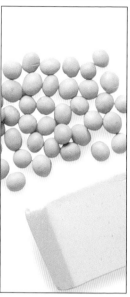

What It Does: Necessary for the growth and maintenance of bones, teeth, and healthy gums; maintains normal blood pressure normal; may reduce risk of heart disease; enables muscles, including the heart, to contract; is essential for normal blood clotting; needed for proper nerve impulse transmission; maintains connective tissue; helps prevent rickets and osteoporosis.

Minimum Recommended Daily Allowance: Adults, 800 mg; pregnant women, 1,200 mg.

Food Sources: Asparagus, cruciferous vegetables, dairy products, dark leafy vegetables, figs, legumes, nuts, oats, prunes, salmon with bones, sardines with bones, seeds, soybeans, tempeh, tofu.

Toxic Dosage: Daily intake of 2,000 mg or more can lead to constipation, calcium deposits in the soft tissue, urinary tract infections, and possible interference with the body's absorption of zinc.

Enemies: Alcohol, caffeine, excessive sugar intake, high-protein diet, high sodium intake, inadequate levels of vitamin D, soft drinks containing phosphorous.

Deficiency Symptoms: Aching joints, brittle nails, eczema, elevated blood cholesterol. heart palpitations, hypertension, insomnia, muscle cramps, nervousness, pallor, tooth decay.

IRON

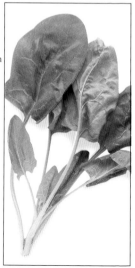

What It Does: Aids in the production of hemoglobin (the protein in red blood cells that transports oxygen from the lungs to the body's tissue) and myoglobin (a protein that provides extra fuel to muscles during exertion); helps maintain healthy immune system; is important for growth.

Minimum Recommended Daily Allowance: Men, 10 mg; women, 15 mg; pregnant women, 30 mg.

Food Sources: Beef, blackstrap molasses, brewer's yeast, dark green vegetables, dried fruit, legumes, nuts, organ meats, sea vegetables, seeds, soybeans, tempeh, whole grains.

Toxic Dosage: Iron should not be taken in excess of 35 mg daily without a doctor's recommendation. In high doses, iron cam cause diarrhea, dizziness, fatigue, headaches, stomach-aches, weakened pulse. Excess iron inhibits the absorption of phosphorus and vitamin E, interferes with immune function, and has been associated with cancer, cirrhosis, heart disease.

Enemies: Antacids, caffeine, tetracycline, iron absorption, excessive menstrual bleeding, long-term illness, an ulcer.

Deficiency Symptoms: Anemia, brittle hair, difficulty swallowing, dizziness, fatigue, hair loss, irritability, nervousness, pallor, ridges on the nails, sensitivity to cold, slowed mental reactions.

MAGNESIUM

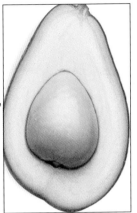

What It Does: Plays a role in formation of bone; protects arterial linings from stress caused by sudden blood pressure; helps body metabolize carbohydrates and minerals; assists in building proteins; helps maintain healthy bones and teeth; reduces one's risk of developing osteoporosis.

Minimum Recommended Daily Allowance: Men, 350 mg; women, 280 mg; pregnant women, 320 mg.

Food Sources: Apples, apricots, avocados, bananas, blackstrap molasses, brewer's yeast. brown rice, cantaloupe, dairy products, figs, garlic, green leafy vegetables, legumes, nuts.

Toxic Dosage: Daily doses over 3,000 mg can lead to diarrhea, fatigue, muscle weakness, and in extreme cases, severely depressed heart rate and blood pressure, shallow breathing, loss of reflexes and coma.

Enemies: Alcohol, diuretics, high-fat intake, high-protein diet.

Deficiency Symptoms: Though deficiency is rare, symptoms include disorientation, heart palpitations, listlessness, muscle weakness.

POTASSIUM

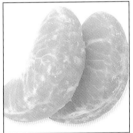

What It Does: Maintains a healthy nervous system and regular heart rhythm; helps prevent stroke; aids in proper muscle contractions; controls the body's water balance; assists chemical reactions within cells; aids in the transmission of electrochemical impulses; maintains stable blood pressure; required for protein synthesis, carbohydrate metabolism, and insulin secretion by the pancreas.

Minimum Recommended Daily Allowance: Adults, 2,000 mg.

Food Sources: Apricots, avocados, bananas, blackstrap molasses, brewer's yeast, brown rice, citrus fruits, dairy.

Toxic Dosage: Should not be taken in excess of 18 grams.

Enemies: Diarrhea, diuretics, caffeine use, heavy perspiration, kidney disorders, tobacco use.

Deficiency Symptoms: Chills, dry skin, constipation, depression, diminished reflexes, edema, headaches, insatiable thirst, fluctuations in heartbeat, nervousness, respiratory distress.

ZINC

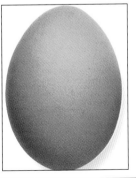

What It Does: Contributes to a wide range of bodily processes. Aids in cell respiration; assists in bone development; helps energy metabolism, promotes wound healing; regulates heart rate and blood pressure; helps liver remove toxic substances, such as alcohol, from the body.

Minimum Recommended Daily Allowance: Adults, 15 mg; pregnant women, 30 mg.

Food Sources: Brewer's yeast, cheese, egg yolks, lamb, legumes, mushrooms, nuts, organ meats, sea food, sea vegetables, seeds.

Toxic Dosage: Do not take more than 100 mg of zinc daily. In doses this high, zinc can depress the immune system.

Deficiency Symptoms: Appetite loss, dermatitis, fatigue, impaired wound healing, loss of taste, white streaks on the nails.

INDEX

ABOUT THE AUTHOR

Stephanie Pedersen is a writer and editor who specializes in the area of health. Her articles have appeared in numerous publications, including *American Woman, Sassy, Teen, Weight Watchers* and *Woman's World*. She has also co-written *What Your Cat is Trying to Tell You: A Head-to-Tail Guide to Your Cat's Symptoms and Their Solutions* and *What Your Dog is Trying to Tell You: A Head-to-Tail Guide to Your Dog's Symptoms and Their Solutions*, both published by St. Martin's Press. She currently resides in New York City.

Picture Credits: Steve Gorton, David Murray, Dave King, Martin Norris, Philip Gatward, Andy Crawford, Philip Dowell, Clive Streeter, Peter Chadwick, Tim Ridley, Andrew Whittack, Martin Cameron

DORLING KINDERSLEY PUBLISHING, INC.
www.dk.com

Published in the United States by
Dorling Kindersley Publishing, Inc.
95 Madison Avenue • New York, New York 10016

Editorial Director: LaVonne Carlson
Editors: Nancy Burke, Barbara Minton, Connie Robinson
Designer: Carol Wells
Cover Designer: Gus Yoo

Library of Congress Cataloging-in-Publication Data is available upon request.
ISBN: 0-7894-5197-2

First American Edition   10 9 8 7 6 5 4 3 2 1